MW00980088

WEIGHT LOSS:
60 DELICIOUS KETOGENIC DIET RECIPES

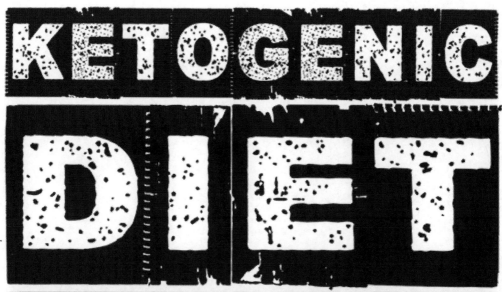

KETOGENIC DIET

60 MOUTHWATERING MEALS

1 MONTH OF LOW-CARB, HIGH-FAT WEIGHT LOSS MEALS

Recipes365

Copyright © 2016

Recipes 365

All rights reserved. No part of this publication may be reproduced, distributed, or transmitted in any form or by any means, including photocopying, recording, or other electronic or mechanical methods, without the prior written permission of the publisher, except in the case of brief quotations embodied in critical reviews and certain other non-commercial uses permitted by copyright law.

• BEFORE YOU BEGIN •

Free Bonus Guide:

Top 10 Ketogenic Diet Mistakes

We've put together a free companion guide to go with this recipe book. It features the top 10 mistakes made by people on the ketogenic diet.

If you want to avoid costly mistakes and accelerate your progress you will find a link below to get it below now!

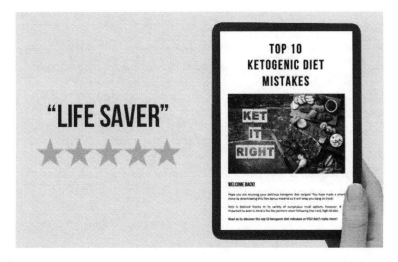

Visit www.litomedia.com/ketogenic-mistakes to get your free bonus guide!

Table of Contents

Dinners

Desserts

"One cannot think well, love well, sleep well, if one has not dined well."

-Virginia Woolf

INTRODUCTION

Welcome to the world's most effective high-fat, low-carb diet! By now you are probably well aware of the benefits of going keto, but just in case you need to refresh your memory here's a quick top-up before we dive into the recipes.

THE SCIENCE IN A NUTSHELL

Your body normally converts carbohydrates into glucose for energy. By limiting your intake and replacing it with fats, your body enters a state of ketosis.

Here your body produces ketones, created by a breakdown of fats in the liver. Without carbohydrates as your primary source of energy your body will turn to the ketones instead.

This effectively cranks up the fat burning furnace and puts your body in the ultimate metabolic state.

WHAT KETO CAN DO FOR YOU

Keto has its origins in treating healthcare conditions such as epilepsy, diabetes, cardiovascular disease, metabolic syndrome, auto-brewery syndrome and high blood pressure but now has much wider application in weight control.

This diet, then, will take you above and beyond typical results and propel you into a new realm of total body health. If you want to look and feel the best you possibly can, all without sacrificing your love of delicious food, then this is the cookbook for you.

THINGS TO REMEMBER

A good diet is not solution to anything in and of itself; it must be applied as part of a healthy lifestyle in order to see maximum results.

Think of the ketogenic diet as the foundation for your new body. If you want to build something truly special on top of it then design your lifestyle with that goal in mind.

Cutting out junk food goes without saying, as does ditching bad habits such as smoking and drinking. Exercise, too, will take you to heights you never knew were possible.

So, as you explore these delectable dishes and embark on the keto diet, try not to neglect other areas or responsibility.

We recommend getting some professional advice from a physician prior to commencing, since they will be able to advise you much better on your own individual goals.

With that said, we just know you will love every bite of what's to come. Don't forget to share the love and tell a friend. Having them with you on this journey will be incredibly motivational.

This is the start of something great. Let's go!

THE RECIPES

We wanted to make it as simple as possible for you to get in the kitchen and rustle up something special, so you will find each recipe laid out in an easy to follow format.

Each begins with a short intro to the dish, followed by the serving size and list of ingredients. Remember, this diet is designed to rekindle your love of food, not extinguish it with rules and regulations, so don't be afraid to experiment.

Use the ingredients as general guidelines and follow the instructions as best you can. You may not get everything perfect first time, every time, but that is what makes it yours!

Cooking and eating shouldn't be about presentation, so you won't find any fancy pictures here. In fact, you won't find any pictures at all, because they will just distract you from your goals.

When you obsess over replicating recipes to the exact photographic standards of a professional chef it becomes an impossible task. Instead, simply follow the recipes and find your own rhythm. Soon enough, you'll have created your own signature dishes!

Each recipe ends with a breakdown of key nutritional information including number of calories and amount of fats, carbohydrates and protein.

Again, this isn't to be obsessed over. Food is something to be enjoyed, so don't go trying to calculate your macros to four decimal points! Be responsible when monitoring your progress, but be reasonable, too.

Once you start loving what you are eating mealtimes will become something to look forward to, and that's when the magic happens.

So without further ado, go forth, and cook to your heart's content!

"One cannot think well, love well, sleep well, if one has not dined well."

-Virginia Woolf

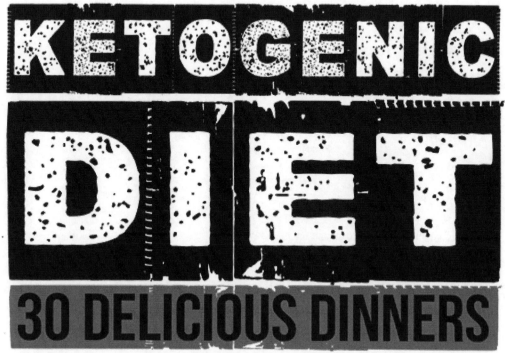

30 DELICIOUS DINNERS

1 MONTH OF LOW-CARB, HIGH-FAT WEIGHT LOSS MEALS

Recipes365

Nutty Salmon

This walnut crust salmon is sure to be a hit for dinner. Deliciously seasoned with mustard and dill, and it's packed with healthy fats to keep you on your diet.

SERVING SIZE:
This recipe yields 2 servings.

INGREDIENTS:

1/4 tsp. dill

1 tbsp. olive oil

1 tbsp. dijon mustard

2 salmon fillets (3 oz. each)

1/2 cup walnuts

2 tbsp. maple syrup (sugar free)

Salt and pepper to taste

DIRECTIONS:

1. Preheat your oven to 350°F.

2. Dump your syrup, mustard, and walnuts into a blender or food processor.

3. Pulse until you have a paste.

4. Heat a stovetop pan on high. Once hot, place your salmon skin side down in the pan.

5. Sear the salmon for about 3 minutes until the skin is crisp.

6. While searing the skin side, add the walnut paste to the side facing up.

7. Once done searing, transfer to the oven and bake for 7 to 8 minutes.

All done, enjoy!

NUTRITIONAL INFORMATION (PER SERVING):

Calories: 375

Fat: 44g

Carbs: 4g

Protein: 22g

CROCK POT OXTAILS

The crock pot is your best friend for dinner on a busy schedule. Just toss in the ingredients, forget for a few hours, and you've got a wonderful hot meal all ready. One such recipe is this crock pot oxtails dish.

SERVING SIZE:

This recipe yields 3 servings.

INGREDIENTS:

1 tsp. onion powder

3 tbsp. tomato paste

1 tsp. garlic (minced)

1 tbsp. fish sauce

2 tbsp. soy sauce

1 tsp. thyme (dried)

1/2 tsp. ginger (ground)

1/3 cup butter

2 lbs. oxtails

2 cups beef broth

1/2 tsp. guar gum

Salt and pepper to taste

DIRECTIONS:

1. Heat the beef broth on the stove, then add the fish sauce, tomato paste, soy sauce, and butter.

2. Once fully heated and mixed, add the mixture to a slow cooker and season with all your spices.

3. Add the oxtails to the slow cooker and mix well.

4. Set the slow cooker on low, and let cook for 7 hours.

5. Remove just the oxtails from the slow cooker, and set aside.

6. Now add the guar gum to what remains in the slow cooker, and use an immersion blender to pulse your mixture.

7. Now serve your oxtails and sauce along with your favorite side dish.

Enjoy!

NUTRITIONAL INFORMATION (PER SERVING):

Calories; 430

Fat: 30g

Carbs: 3.5g

Protein: 29g

KETO ASIAN STYLE SHORT RIBS

Give your standard ribs a delightful twist by throwing in some Asian style spice! The combination of ginger, soy sauce, and red pepper give this recipe a wonderful kick.

SERVING SIZE:

This recipe yields 4 servings.

INGREDIENTS:

Ribs and Marinade:

2 tbsp. rice vinegar

1/4 cup soy sauce

2 tbsp. fish sauce

6 large short ribs, flank cut (about 1.5 lbs.)

Asian Spice:

1/2 tsp. red pepper flakes

1/2 tsp. garlic (minced)

1/2 tsp. onion powder

1 tsp. ginger (ground)

1/2 tsp. sesame seed

1 tbsp. salt

1/4 tsp. cardamom

DIRECTIONS:

1. For the ribs, mix all of the marinade ingredients. Marinade the ribs for at least an hour.

2. Mix together all of the ingredients for the spice rub.

3. Remove the ribs from the marinade and rub with the spices from the previous step.

4. Heat your grill, and grill for approximately 5 minutes per side.

Bon appetite!

NUTRITIONAL INFORMATION (PER SERVING):

Calories: 415

Fat: 32g

Carbs: 1g

Protein: 30g

EASY PEEZY PIZZA

When you get home after a long day what can be better than a quick homemade pizza? With a crust of mostly egg and cheese, this keto pizza is delicious and customizable with all your favorite toppings!

SERVING SIZE:

This recipe yields 1 serving.

INGREDIENTS:

Crust:

1/2 tsp. Italian seasoning

1 tbsp. psyllium husk powder

2 large eggs

2 tsp. frying oil of choice

2 tbsp. parmesan cheese

Salt to taste

Toppings:

3 tbsp. tomato sauce

1 tbsp. basil (chopped)

1.5 oz. mozzarella cheese

DIRECTIONS:

1. Use a food processor, or blender, or immersion blender to combine all of the pizza crust ingredients.

2. Heat the oil in a frying pan, and add the crust mixture to the pan when hot. Spread into a circle.

3. Once the edges of the crust begin to brown, flip and cook for an additional 60 seconds.

4. Now top the crust with the cheese and tomato sauce, and broil for 2 minutes until the cheese begins to bubble.

Top with basil and enjoy!

NUTRITIONAL INFORMATION (PER SERVING):

Calories: 460

Fat: 36g

Carbs: 4g

Protein: 28g

SEARED RIBEYE

Ribeye, plain and simple. Just follow the recipe for searing and combine with your favorite fatty side dishes for a perfect keto friendly dinner!

SERVING SIZE:

This recipe yields 3 servings.

INGREDIENTS:

3 tbsp. bacon fat

salt and pepper to taste

2 medium ribeye steaks (about 1.25 lbs.)

DIRECTIONS:

1. Preheat your oven to 250°F.

2. Season the steaks with salt and pepper, then place on wire racks for baking.

3. Insert a meat thermometer into the streak.

4. Bake until the thermometer shows a temperature of 124°F.

5. Now heat a cast iron skillet on the stove and add your bacon grease. When very hot, sear your steaks for about 40 seconds per side.

All set, go eat!

NUTRITIONAL INFORMATION (PER SERVING):

Calories: 425

Fat: 32g

Carbs: 0g

Protein: 31g

KETO SALMON AND DILL SAUCE

The dill and salmon yields a delectable dish with the deep taste of salmon and a slight tangy hint of dill or sharp mustard. Give this salmon and dill sauce recipe a try and see for yourself!

SERVING SIZE:

This recipe yields 2 servings.

INGREDIENTS:

Salmon:

1 tbsp. duck fat

1 tsp. tarragon (dried)

1 tsp. dill weed (dried)

1 1/2 lbs. salmon fillet

Salt and pepper to taste.

Dill Sauce:

1/2 tsp. dill weed (dried)

1/4 cup heavy cream

1/2 tarragon (dried)

2 tbsp. butter

salt and pepper to taste

DIRECTIONS:

1. Slice your salmon so you have two fillets.

2. Season the meaty side with all of your salmon spices, and season the skin side with salt and pepper.

3. Heat a skillet over medium, and add the duck fat. When hot, add the salmon with the skin down.

4. Cook for about 5 minutes as the skin crisps. Once the skin is crispy, flip the salmon and reduce heat to low.

5. Cook for about 10 minutes, or until it is cooked to your liking.

6. When the salmon is removed from the pan, toss in all your spices for the dill sauce, and stir until they begin to turn brown.

7. Add the cream, and stir until hot.

Serve it up!

NUTRITIONAL INFORMATION (PER SERVING):

Calories: 465

Fat: 42g

Carbs: 2g

Protein: 23g

ORANGE DUCK BREAST

Give your duck some tang by mixing in some orange extract. A fun twist on the traditional duck roast, and sure to be an excellent dinner!

SERVING SIZE:

This recipe yields 1 serving.

INGREDIENTS:

1/2 tsp. orange extract

1 tbsp. swerve sweetener

1/4 tsp. sage

1 tbsp. heavy cream

2 tbsp. butter

1 cup spinach

6 oz. duck breast

DIRECTIONS:

1. Season the entire duck breast with salt and pepper, and score the top.

2. Heat a pan over medium-low, and add the butter and swerve. Cook until the butter begins to brown.

3. Add the orange extract and sage. Cook until the butter turns deep amber in color.

4. While this is cooking, set another pan on the stove and heat over medium-high. Add the duck breast to this pan.

5. Cook for a few minutes, or until the skin turns crisp. Then flip.

6. Now add the heavy cream to the butter mixture, and mix well.

7. When hot, pour the mixture over the duck breast, and cook for a further few minutes.

8. Toss the spinach into the pan and cook until wilted.

Enjoy!

NUTRITIONAL INFORMATION (PER SERVING)

Calories: 795

Fat: 72g

Carbs: 0g

Protein: 38g

CLASSIC RIBEYE

Steak, butter, and duck fat. That's all you need for this delicious ribeye along with some thyme for garnish. Try it with your favorite side dishes and enjoy!

SERVING SIZE:

This recipe yields 2 servings.

INGREDIENTS:

1 ribeye steak (~16 oz.)

1 tbsp. butter

1 tbsp. duck fat

1/2 tsp. thyme

Salt and pepper to taste

DIRECTIONS:

1. Preheat your oven to 400°F.

2. Place a cast iron skillet in the oven as it is warming.

3. Once the oven is up to temperature, remove the pan and place on the stove over medium heat.

4. Add the oil and steak to the pan. Sear the steak for about 2 minute

5. Turn over the steak, and bake in the oven for about 5 minutes.

6. Again remove the pan, and place over low heat on the stove.

7. Add your butter and thyme to the pan and mix with the oil.

8. Baste the steak for 4 minutes.

9. Let the steak rest for 5 minutes.

Put it into your face!

NUTRITIONAL INFORMATION (PER SERVING):

Calories: 748

Fat: 65g

Carbs: 0g

Protein: 39g

Chili Turkey Legs

Give those turkey legs some spice by adding chili powder and cayenne pepper! This recipe is easy to follow and will provide you with a tasty and zippy end to your day.

Serving Size:

This recipe yields 4 servings.

Ingredients:

1/2 tsp. onion powder

1 tsp. liquid smoke

1/2 tsp. thyme (dried)

1/2 tsp. pepper

2 tsp. salt

1/4 tsp. cayenne pepper

1/2 tsp. garlic powder

1 tsp. Worcestershire sauce

1/2 tsp. ancho chili powder

2 turkey legs (about 1 lbs. each without bone)

2 tbsp. duck fat

DIRECTIONS:

1. Combine all dry spices in a bowl, then toss in the wet ingredients and mix thoroughly.

2. Dry the turkey legs with paper towel, and then rub in the seasoning.

3. Preheat oven to 350°F.

4. Heat a pan over medium-high, and add the duck fat.

5. When the oil begins to smoke, add the turkey legs and sear for 1 to 2 minutes per side.

6. Bake in the oven for 55 to 60 minutes or until completely cooked.

That's all folks!

NUTRITIONAL INFORMATION (PER SERVING):

Calories: 380

Fat: 21g

Carbs: 0.5g

Protein: 44g

Slow Roasted Pork Shoulder

A hearty roasted pork shoulder to round off the day. Simple preparation, keto friendly, and excellent for entertaining!

Serving Size:

This recipe yields 20 servings.

Ingredients:

1 tsp. black pepper

2 tsp. oregano

1 tsp. onion powder

1 tsp. garlic powder

3 1/2 tsp. salt

8 lbs. pork shoulder

DIRECTIONS:

1. Preheat oven to 250°F.

2. Dry the pork, then rub with the salt and spices.

3. Place the shoulder on a wire rack (a foiled baking sheet works too), and bake for 8 to 10 hours. Or until your meat thermometer reads 190°F.

4. Remove from the oven, and raise oven temperature to 500°F.

5. Cover the shoulder with foil and let rest for about 15 minutes.

6. Remove the foil from the shoulder, and roast in the oven for another 20 minutes, while rotating every 5 minutes.

7. Remove from oven and let rest for 20 minutes.

Serve this bad boy up!

Nutritional information (per serving):

Calories: 460

Fat: 35g

Carbs: 0.5g

Protein: 32g

Asian Spiced Chicken Thighs

Liven up your chicken thighs with some sriracha and red pepper! These zippy little devils provide an excellent laid-back dinner, or a quick snack during the day!

Serving size:
This recipe yields 4 servings.

Ingredients:
1 tsp. ginger (minced)

1 tsp. garlic (minced)

1/4 tsp. xanthan gum

1 tsp. red pepper flakes

1 tbsp. ketchup (sugar free)

1 tbsp. olive oil

1 tbsp. rice wine vinegar

2 tsp. sriracha

4 cups spinach

6 chicken thighs (bone in and skin on)

Salt and pepper to taste

DIRECTIONS:

1. Preheat your oven to 425°F.

2. Dry your chicken and season the skin with salt and pepper.

3. Mix all of the sauce ingredients until a paste begins to form

4. Rub this sauce all over the chicken.

5. Lay the chicken on a wire rack

6. Bake for 45 to 50 minutes, or until the skin is crisp and slight charring appears.

7. Mix the spinach, some salt and pepper, red pepper flakes, and leftover chicken fat together, and serve alongside the baked chicken.

Enjoy!

NUTRITIONAL INFORMATION (PER SERVING):

Calories: 600

Fat: 52g

Carbs: 2g

Protein: 30g

BAKED POBLANO PEPPERS

Very similar to baked stuffed mushrooms, these peppers combine pork, mushrooms, cumin, and chili powder for a delicious dinner!

SERVING SIZE:
This recipe yields 4 servings.

INGREDIENTS:
7 baby bella mushrooms

1/2 onion

1/4 cup cilantro

4 poblano peppers

1 tsp. chili powder

1 tsp. cumin

1 tomato

1 tbsp. bacon fat

1 lb. ground pork

Salt and pepper to taste

DIRECTIONS:

1. Broil your poblano peppers in the oven for about 10 minutes. Flip or move every couple minutes to keep broiling consistent.

2. Heat a pan on the stove, and add the bacon fat. Once browned, add the cumin, chili, salt, and pepper.

3. Dice the onion and toss into the mixture, along with the garlic. Fully mix, and then add the mushrooms

4. Once the mushrooms are cooked, add the cilantro and chopped tomato.

5. Cook for a further 3 minutes.

6. Stuff the poblanos with the mixture and bake at 350°F for 9 to 10 minutes.

You're all done!

NUTRITIONAL INFORMATION (PER SERVING):

Calories: 365

Fat: 28g

Carbs: 6g

Protein: 22g

Coconut Shrimp

Shrimp with a tropical flair! Coconut crusted with a fruity apricot sauce, this keto recipe will fill you up for dinner and also keep those sweet cravings in check.

SERVING SIZE:

This recipe yields 3 servings.

INGREDIENTS:

Shrimp:

1 cup coconut flakes (unsweetened)

2 large egg whites

1 lb. shrimp (peeled and deveined)

2 tbsp. coconut flour

Sauce:

1 tbsp. lime juice

1 1/2 tbsp. rive wine vinegar

1 medium red chili (diced)

1/2 apricot preserves (sugar free)

1/4 tsp. red pepper flakes

DIRECTIONS:

1. Preheat your oven to 400°F

2. Beat the egg whites until soft peaks form.

3. Dip the shrimp in the coconut flour, then dip in the egg whites, then dip in the coconut flakes.

4. Lay the dipped shrimp on a greased baking sheet.

5. Bake the shrimp for 15 minutes

6. Finish them off with a 3 to 5 minute broil to give them some browning.

7. Combine all of the ingredients for the sauce and mix well.

Serve them up and enjoy!

NUTRITIONAL INFORMATION (PER SERVING):

Calories: 395

Fat: 22g

Carbs: 7g

Protein: 37g

SLOW COOKED LAMB

Break out that slow cooker for this fantastic leg of lamb stuffed with savory herbs. Get it prepared in just a few minutes and let the cooker do the rest!

SERVING SIZE:
This recipe yields 6 servings

INGREDIENTS:
3/4 tsp. rosemary (dried)

6 leaves mint

1 tbsp. maple syrup

2 tbsp. whole grain mustard

3/4 tsp. garlic

1/4 cup olive oil

2 lbs. leg of lamb

Salt and pepper to taste

4 sprigs thyme

DIRECTIONS:

1. Cut three slits across the top of the lamb.

2. Heat a slow cooker to low, and rub the lamb with olive oil, syrup, mustard, salt, and pepper.

3. Stuff each slit on the lamb with garlic and rosemary

4. Add to the slow cooker and leave for 7 hours.

5. Add thyme and mint to slow cooker and leave for an additional hour.

Enjoy!

NUTRITIONAL INFORMATION (PER SERVING):

Calories: 415

Fat: 35g

Carbs: 0.5g

Protein: 27g

CHICKEN WITH PAPRIKA

This keto chicken recipe combines sweet and spicy in the form of maple syrup and paprika. Cook this savory chicken in its sauce then drizzle right before serving.

SERVING SIZE:

This recipe yields 4 servings.

INGREDIENTS:

2 tbsp. Spanish smoked paprika

3 tbsp. olive oil

1 tbsp. maple syrup

2 tbsp. lemon juice

2 tsp. garlic (minced)

4 chicken breasts (boneless and skinless)

Salt and pepper to taste

DIRECTIONS:

1. Preheat your oven to 350°F.

2. Cut the chicken into chunks and season with the salt and pepper.

3. Combine all other ingredients separately to make the sauce.

4. Add about 1/3 of the sauce to your baking casserole dish or pan. Lay chicken on top of sauce.

5. Drizzle the rest of the sauce over the chicken.

6. Bake for 30 to 35 minutes, and then broil for a further 5 minutes.

Serve!

NUTRITIONAL INFORMATION (PER SERVING):

Calories: 275

Fat: 13.5g

Carbs: 2.5g

Protein: 36.5g

CURRIED CHICKEN THIGHS

A straight forward, keto friendly method for whipping up some curried chicken. Easy to cook and excellent for those tired weeknights!

SERVING SIZE:

This recipe yields 8 servings.

INGREDIENTS:

1/2 tsp. chili powder

1/2 tsp. coriander (ground)

1/2 tsp. cinnamon (ground)

1/2 tsp. cayenne pepper

1/2 tsp. allspice

1/2 tsp. cardamom (ground)

1/4 tsp. ginger

1 tsp. cumin (ground)

1 tsp. paprika

1 tsp. garlic powder

2 tsp. yellow curry

8 chicken thighs (bone in and skin on)

1/4 cup olive oil

1 1/2 tsp. salt

DIRECTIONS:

1. Preheat oven to 425°F.

2. In a bowl, mix all of your spices together.

3. Line a baking sheet with foil, and place all the chicken on the foil.

4. Rub the olive oil and spices over the chicken.

5. Bake for 50 minutes are until completely cooked.

6. Cool for 5 to 8 minutes.

Go enjoy your evening!

NUTRITIONAL INFORMATION (PER SERVING):

Calories: 278

Fat: 20g

Carbs: 0.5g

Protein: 22g

APPLEWOOD PORK CHOPS

Give your pork chops a subtle hint of Applewood and delicious dinner is all yours! Combine with your favorite fatty side dish and you've an excellent keto meal right in front of you.

SERVING SIZE:

This recipe yields 4 servings.

INGREDIENTS:

1/2 tsp. garlic powder

1 tsp. grill mates Applewood rub

1/2 tsp. black pepper

1/2 tsp. Mrs. Dash (table blend)

1 tsp. salt

2 tbsp. olive oil

2 2tsp. hidden valley powdered ranch

4 pork chops (bone in)

DIRECTIONS:

1. Combine all of the spices and rub into the pork chops.

2. Heat a pan on medium, and add the olive oil.

3. When hot, add the pork chops and cover.

4. Cook for about 10 minutes and then flip the chops.

5. Cook for a further 5 minutes (covered).

6. Turn the heat up to high, and flip chops again. Keep the pan uncovered now.

7. Cook for 2 minutes, and then let rest for 4 minutes

Serve and enjoy!

NUTRITIONAL INFORMATION (PER SERVING):

Calories: 260

Fat: 13g

Carbs: 1.5g

Protein: 35g

CHICKEN STEW

Whether it's a chilly, rainy, or stormy day; good old fashioned chicken stew is an excellent choice for dinner. Warming and comforting, this recipe fits the bill with some extra zip from hot wing sauce.

SERVING SIZE:
This recipe yields 5 servings.

INGREDIENTS:
2 tsp. garlic (minced)

3 tbsp. butter

2 tsp. paprika

2 tsp. ranch seasoning

1 tsp. red pepper flakes

1 tsp. oregano

1/2 cup sliced tomatoes

1 1/2 tomato sauce

3 lbs. chicken thigh

1 green pepper

1/3 cup hot wing sauce

3 cups mushrooms

DIRECTIONS:

1. Finely slice your mushrooms and pepper.

2. Set your crock pot on high and add the thighs, tomato slices, garlic, spices, tomato sauce, and hot sauce.

3. Also toss in peppers and mix.

4. Let the mixture cook for 2 hours.

5. Now turn the pot to low, give the mix a stir, and cook for 4 to 5 hours.

6. Dump in 3 tbsp. of butter and give another stir.

7. Remove the lid, and cook for an hour.

Savor the glory!

NUTRITIONAL INFORMATION (PER SERVING):

Calories: 360

Fat: 22g

Carbs: 8g

Protein: 33g

ASIAN PORK CHOPS

Once again, give the 'old reliable' recipes an upgrade by including some Asian style spices. Here we have pork chops mixed with anise, soy sauce, and sesame oil to create a unique and enjoyable culinary experience.

SERVING SIZE:

This recipe yields 2 servings.

INGREDIENTS:

1/2 tbsp. sambal chili paste

1/2 tsp. five spice

1/2 tbsp. ketchup (sugar free)

1 stalk lemon grass

4 garlic cloves (halved)

1 tbsp. almond flour

1 tbsp. fish sauce

1/2 tsp. peppercorns

1 1/2 tsp. soy sauce

1 tsp. sesame oil

1 medium star anise

4 boneless pork chops

DIRECTIONS:

1. Pound the pork chops to 1/2 inch thickness

2. Grind the peppercorns and star anise to a fine powder.

3. Combine the pepper, anise, lemongrass, and garlic. Grind until a paste forms.

4. Marinade the chops with the paste

5. Let the chops marinate for about 2 hours at room temperature.

6. Heat a pan on high. Coat your pork chops with the almond flour.

7. Sear the chops in the pan. This should take about 1 to 2 minutes per side.

8. Once the pork is cooked, cut them into slices.

9. Mix the sambal and ketchup to create your sauce.

Enjoy your masterpiece!

NUTRITIONAL INFORMATION (PER SERVING):

Calories: 275

Fat: 10g

Carbs: 5g

Protein: 35g

PORTOBELLO BURGERS

The constant battle to avoid the carbs in bread can be draining. But you can still have a good old fashioned burger! Dive into this recipe with the twist of mushrooms for the buns.

SERVING SIZE:

This recipe yields 1 serving.

INGREDIENTS:

Bun:

1 tsp. oregano

1 clove garlic

1/2 tbsp. coconut oil

2 Portobello mushroom caps

1 pinch each of salt and pepper

Burger:

1 tsp. each of salt and pepper

6 oz. beef

1 tbsp. dijon mustard

1/4 cup cheddar cheese

DIRECTIONS:

1. Preheat a griddle on high

2. In a container, combine the oil and spices for the bun

3. Scrape out the insides of the mushrooms, and marinate in the oil and spices

4. In a separate bowl, combine the meat, salt, pepper, cheese, and mustard.

5. Use your hands to form your burger patties.

6. Now add your mushrooms to the griddle and cook about 8 minutes.

7. Remove the mushrooms and toss the patties on. Cook about 5 minutes per side.

8. Assemble your burger with whatever toppings you like.

That's it!

NUTRITIONAL INFORMATION (PER SERVING):

Calories: 730

Fat: 46g

Carbs: 5g

Protein: 62g

BBQ Chicken Pizza

Slash the carbs in your pizza by making your own crust out of eggs and cheese! This recipe for BBQ chicken pizza will guide you through the quick and painless process of making your own pizza crust, along with some delectable toppings.

SERVING SIZE:

This recipe yields 4 servings.

INGREDIENTS:

Crust:

1 1/2 tsp. Italian seasoning

6 tbsp. parmesan cheese

3 tbsp. psyllium husk powder

6 large eggs

salt and pepper to taste

Toppings:

1 tbsp. mayonnaise

4 tbsp. tomato sauce

6 oz. rotisserie chicken (shredded)

4 tbsp. BBQ sauce

4 oz. cheddar cheese

DIRECTIONS:

1. Pre heat your oven to 425°F.

2. Combine all ingredients for the crust in a blender and pulse until thick. An immersion blender will serve this purpose as well.

3. Now spread the dough into a circle on a baking sheet or oven stone. Be sure you grease the surface first.

4. Bake for 10 minutes.

5. Flip the crust over, and pile up your toppings.

6. Broil for a further 10 minutes.

Enjoy, you deserve it.

NUTRITIONAL INFORMATION (PER SERVING):

Calories: 355

Fat: 25g

Carbs: 3g

Protein: 25g

CHEESE STUFFED BURGER

Imagine taking a bit from a juicy burger, and suddenly, there's cheese! The cheese stuffed burger, or the Juicy Lucy, is sure to be a grill or dinnertime favorite.

SERVING SIZE:
This recipe yields 2 servings / burgers.

INGREDIENTS:
1 oz. mozzarella cheese

1/2 tsp. pepper

1 tsp salt

2 oz. cheddar cheese

1 tsp. Cajun seasoning

1 tbsp. butter

2 slices bacon (cooked)

8 oz. ground beef

DIRECTIONS:

1. Use your hands to work all the spices into the beef.

2. Form your patties with the mozzarella cheese stuffed inside

3. Heat a pan on the stove and add 1 tbsp. of butter. When hot, add burger to the pan and cover.

4. Cook 2 to 3 minutes, flip, and sprinkle cheese on top. Cover again and cook to taste.

5. Feel fresh to recharge the butter in between burgers if you wish.

6. Chop your bacon and top the burgers.

Voila, ready to go!

NUTRITIONAL INFORMATION (PER SERVING):

Calories: 612

Fat: 50g

Carbs: 2g

Protein: 32g

TATER TOT STYLE NACHOS

What happens when you combine two cheesy side dishes? You get one amazingly delicious dinner course! This recipe for tater tot nachos tastes just as good as it sounds.

SERVING SIZE:

This recipe yields 2 servings.

INGREDIENTS:

6 oz. ground beef (cooked)

2 tbsp. sour cream

6 black olives

1 tbsp. salsa

1/2 jalapeno (sliced)

2 oz. cheddar cheese

2 tater tots (preferably homemade)

DIRECTIONS:

1. In a small cast iron skillet (or casserole dish) place 10 tots as the base layer.

2. Now add half of your beef and cheddar cheese. Repeat this stack-up again until you use all your ingredients.

3. Broil the dish for about 5 minutes until the cheese is fully melted and bubbly.

4. Serve with the black olives, sour cream, and jalapenos.

Enjoy!

NUTRITIONAL INFORMATION (PER SERVING):

Calories: 635

Fat: 53g

Carbs: 6g

Protein: 30g

CHIPOTLE CHICKEN WINGS WITH BLACKBERRY JAM

Game day for your favorite team? Have to bring food to a get together? Then whip up these tasty chipotle style chicken wings! Great for sharing or keep them all to yourself, and the blackberry jam in the next recipe makes the perfect side.

SERVING SIZE:

This recipe yields 5 servings

INGREDIENTS:

1/2 cup chipotle jam with blackberries (see next recipe)

1/2 cup water

3 lbs. chicken wings (~20)

Salt and pepper to taste

DIRECTIONS:

1. Combine the jam and water in a bowl using a fork or whisk to make sure everything is well mixed.

2. In a plastic bag, add all of the chicken, about 2/3s of the jam, salt, and pepper to taste. Make sure everything is well combined and leave to marinate for at least an hour.

3. Preheat oven to 400°F.

4. Lay the chicken on a greased baking sheet, and back for 15 minutes.

5. Flip the chicken, crank the temperature to 425°F, spread the remaining sauce over top, and back for another 25 to 30 minutes.

Eat as is or add the next recipe in.

NUTRITIONAL INFORMATION (PER SERVING):

Calories: 500

Fat: 40g

Carbs: 1.5g

Protein: 35g

CHIPOTLE JAM WITH BLACKBERRY

The spicy and fruity combination in this chipotle style blackberry jam makes this sauce an excellent accompaniment for almost any meat. We recommend dishing it up with our recipe for chipotle chicken wings.

SERVING SIZE:

This recipe yields 10 servings / tablespoons.

INGREDIENTS:

8 drops liquid stevia

1/4 cup MCT oil

1/4 cup erythritol

1/4 tsp. guar gum

8 oz. blackberries

1 1/2 whole chipotle peppers

DIRECTIONS:

1. Heat a pan over low, and add the blackberries. Cook until they are soft and have released their juices.

2. Add everything except the oil and guar gum to the pan. Use a fork to crush the blackberries and mix well.

3. Now turn up the heat to medium, add the oil, and bring to a boil.

4. Once boiling, reduce heat and simmer for a good 8 minutes.

5. Add the guar gum, and mix completely. Using a colander, strain the mixture into a container.

Stick on the side of a dish or eat solo!

NUTRITIONAL INFORMATION (PER SERVING):

Calories: 50

Fat: 6g

Carbs: 1.5g

Protein: 0.5g

JALAPENO SOUP

If you're ready to take a break from the standard savory soups and stews, then give this jalapeno soup a try! Creamy and full of chicken this recipe will satisfy your spicy side (especially if you keep the jalapeno seeds in!)

SERVING SIZE:

This recipe yields 6 servings.

INGREDIENTS:

1 tsp. cilantro (dried)

1 tsp. onion powder

1 tsp. Cajun seasoning

1 tbsp. chicken fat

3 jalapenos (diced)

3 cups chicken broth

4 slices bacon (cooked)

6 oz. cream cheese

4 oz. cheddar cheese

4 chicken thighs (deboned)

salt and pepper to taste

2 tsp. garlic (minced)

DIRECTIONS:

1. Preheat your oven to 400°F.

2. Rub the seasoning onto the chicken and bake for 50 to 55 minutes.

3. Heat a pan over medium-high and add the chicken fat. Once hot, add your chicken bones and fry them for 10 minute.

4. Toss in the garlic and jalapenos. Stir and cook for another 4 minutes.

5. Now pour in the broth and spices. Continue to simmer while the chicken bakes.

6. Remove the chicken skin from the thighs and the bones from the pot.

7. Use an immersion blender to puree the jalapenos and garlic. Shred the meat and add to the pot.

8. Simmer for a further 10 minutes

9. Add the cream cheese and cheddar cheese. Stir to fully incorporate and simmer for 10 more minutes.

Garnish with the bacon and enjoy!

NUTRITIONAL INFORMATION (PER SERVING):

Calories: 550

Fat: 43g

Carbs: 4g

Protein: 34g

BACON CHEDDAR SOUP

When is it not a good time for bacon and cheese? Yup, that's what we thought. So dive into this bacon cheddar soup with gusto and enjoy!

SERVING SIZE:

This recipe yields 5 servings.

INGREDIENTS:

1 tsp. garlic powder

1/2 tsp. celery seed

1 tsp. thyme (dried)

1 tsp. onion powder

3/4 cup heavy cream

1/2 tsp. cumin

3 cups chicken broth

4 tbsp. butter

1/2 lbs. bacon

8 oz. cheddar cheese

Salt and pepper to taste

4 jalapeno peppers (diced)

DIRECTIONS:

1. Chop up the bacon to 1 inch slices. Cook until crisp and save the fat.

2. Now dice your jalapenos and cook in the saved bacon fat.

3. Now toss the bacon fat (we're still using it!) into a pot, along with the butter, spices, and broth. Bring the pot to a boil.

4. Once boiling, reduce heat and simmer for 15 minutes.

5. Use a food processor or immersion blender to puree the mixture. Then add the cream and shredded cheese.

6. Stir everything together and keep simmering. Salt and pepper to taste.

7. Add jalapenos and bacon to the pot and simmer for a final 5 minutes.

Enjoy!

NUTRITIONAL INFORMATION (PER SERVING):

Calories: 520

Fat: 50g

Carbs: 4g

Protein: 20g

KETO CHICKEN NUGGETS

Have a hankering for some fast food chicken nuggets? Then make your own keto version! This recipe will satisfy your craving while still keeping you firmly on the ketogenic diet.

SERVING SIZE:

This recipe yields 4 servings.

INGREDIENTS:

Nuggets:

1/4 tsp. paprika

1/4 tsp. salt

1/4 tsp pepper

1/8 tsp. onion powder

1/8 tsp. cayenne pepper

1/4 tsp. chili powder

1/8 tsp. garlic powder

zest from 1 lime

1/4 cup almond flour

1 large egg

24 oz. chicken thighs

1.5 oz. pork rinds

1/4 cup flax meal

Sauce:

1 tbsp. lime juice

1/8 tsp. cumin

1/4 tsp. garlic powder

1/2 tsp. red chili flakes

1/2 avocado

1/2 cup mayonnaise

DIRECTIONS:

1. Add all the ingredients for the crust to a food processor and pulse together.

2. Put the crumbs in a bowl.

3. Whisk the egg is in separate container.

4. Dip each piece of chicken in the eggs and then crumbles, and lay on a greased baking tray.

5. Heat the oven to 400°F, and back for 15 to 18 minutes.

6. Make the sauce by combining all of the sauce ingredients, and mixing well.

Feast!

NUTRITIONAL INFORMATION (PER SERVING):

Calories: 612

Fat: 49g

Carbs: 2g

Protein: 39g

PORK TACOS

Here's your keto version of the classic pork taco. Pepper, lettuce, and pork and flax seed tortillas; easy to put together and add any other toppings that you feel like!

SERVING SIZE:
This recipe yields 3 servings.

INGREDIENTS:
1/4 tsp. garlic powder

1/4 tsp. oregano

3/4 yellow pepper

1/4 tsp. onion powder

1 lbs. pork shoulder (cooked)

1 tbsp. olive oil

1/2 tsp. salt

1/2 tsp. chipotle powder

1 jalapeno pepper

1 cup romaine lettuce

6 thin flax tortillas

1/4 tsp. pepper

DIRECTIONS:

1. Chop your pork into cubes. You can also shred it if you wish.

2. Combine all spices and oil, and add to plastic bag.

3. Toss the pork into the plastic bag and marinade for at least 45 minutes.

4. Heat 1 tbsp. olive oil in a sauce pan set to high heat; chop the vegetables and add to pan.

5. When vegetables are done, cook the pork on high heat until completely done and crisp.

6. Assemble your tacos with the vegetables, lettuce, and pork

Enjoy!

NUTRITIONAL INFORMATION (PER SERVING):

Calories: 715

Fat: 68g

Carbs: 3.5g

Protein: 36g

CHICKEN DRESSED AS BACON

This chicken can't pull the wool over our eyes; even though it will look like one giant slab of bacon once you wrap your bacon slices around the outside, and then bake it in a remarkable lemon mustard sauce. Sounds good doesn't it?

SERVING SIZE:
This recipe yields 8 servings.

INGREDIENTS:
1 small lime

1 tbsp. grain mustard

1 medium lemon

10 strips bacon

3 lbs. whole chicken (gutted)

4 sprigs fresh thyme

Salt and pepper to taste

DIRECTIONS:

1. Preheat oven to 500°F.

2. Season the chicken with salt and pepper, and stuff with the lemon, lime, and thyme.

3. Season bacon with salt and pepper and wrap over the chicken any way you wish.

4. Add the chicken to a roasting pan, and bake for 15 minutes.

5. Lower temperature to 350°F, and bake for a further 45 minutes.

6. Take the chicken out of the pan and place in foil, and transfer the fat and juice to a stovetop pan.

7. Bring pan to a boil and add mustard. Mix well.

Serve with the sauce on the side!

NUTRITIONAL INFORMATION (PER SERVING):

Calories: 375

Fat: 30g

Carbs: 2g

Protein: 24g

"I like food. I like eating. And I don't want to deprive myself of good food."

-Sarah Michelle Gellar

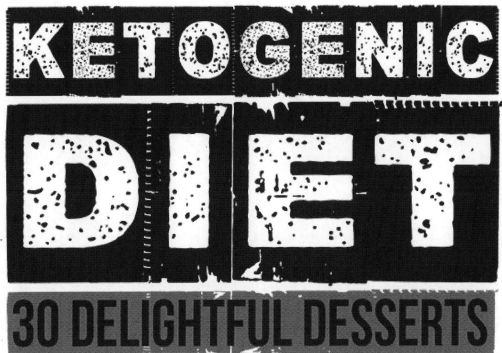

KETOGENIC DIET

30 DELIGHTFUL DESSERTS

1 MONTH OF LOW-CARB, HIGH-FAT WEIGHT LOSS MEALS

Recipes365

COCONUT BARS

These keto no-bake bars are a breeze to make! Just mix everything together and let 'em chill in the fridge.

SERVING SIZE:

This recipe yields 8 servings.

INGREDIENTS:

1 tsp. cinnamon

1/4 cup butter (melted)

1/2 cup cashews

1/4 cup maple syrup (sugar free)

1 cup almond flour

1/4 cup shredded coconut

1 pinch salt

DIRECTIONS:

1. Add the almond flour and melted flour to a large bowl. Mix well.

2. Now (with dramatic flourish) toss in the salt, syrup, coconut, and cinnamon.

3. Roughly chop the cashews and toss into the mixture. Make sure everything is well combined.

4. Place parchment paper in a baking dish and evenly spread the coconut mixture.

Chill for at least 2 hours.

Slice and munch!

NUTRITIONAL INFORMATION (PER SERVING):

Calories: 185

Fat: 18g

Carbs: 4.5g

Protein: 4g

PUMPKIN ICE CREAM WITH PECANS

Ice cream isn't just for the carb carefree anymore! Try the delicious pumpkin, keto friendly, ice cream recipe made with cottage cheese!

SERVING SIZE:

This recipe yields 4 servings.

INGREDIENTS:

2 cups coconut milk

1/2 tsp. xanthan gum

20 drops liquid stevia

1/2 cup pumpkin puree

1/2 cup cottage cheese

1/3 cup erythritol

3 large egg yolks

1 tsp. maple extract

1/2 cup pecans (toasted and chopped)

2 tbsp. butter (Salted)

1 tsp. pumpkin spice

DIRECTIONS:

1. Heat a pan on the stove and toss in the butter and pecans.

2. Now blend the remaining ingredients in either a blender, food processor, or immersion blender.

3. Now add the blended mixture to your ice cream machine, along with the pecans and butter.

4. Follow the churning instructions on your ice cream maker.

Simple as that, go eat!

NUTRITIONAL INFORMATION (PER SERVING):

Calories: 245

Fat: 22g

Carbs: 4g

Protein: 7g

PUMPKIN BLONDIES

These wonderfully soft and fluffy blondies with almond flour, pumpkin, and coconut will be an excellent treat during the day. Or the perfect dish of goodies to bring to a party!

SERVING SIZE:

This recipe yields 12 servings.

INGREDIENTS:

1/2 cup pumpkin puree

1/8 tsp. pumpkin pie spice

1 tsp. maple extract

1/4 cup almond flour

1/2 cup erythritol

1 large egg

1/2 cup butter (softened)

1 tsp. cinnamon

2 tbsp. coconut flour

15 drops liquid stevia

1 oz. pecans (chopped)

DIRECTIONS:

1. Preheat the oven to 350°F.

2. Mix the erythritol, puree, egg, and butter with an electric mixer.

3. Add the flours, cinnamon, stevia, pumpkin pie spice, and maple extract. Run through with the electric mixer again.

4. Grease a brownie pan, preferably with coconut oil, and pour in the mixture.

5. Sprinkle the chopped pecans over top.

6. Bake for about 20 to 25 minutes, until the edges and top appear golden.

Yours to enjoy!

NUTRITIONAL INFORMATION (PER SERVING):

Calories: 110

Fat: 11g

Carbs: 1.5g

Protein: 2g

PEANUT BUTTER FUDGE

Peanut butter? Right here. Fudge? Roger. Dark chocolate? Look no further. This peanut butter fudge recipe is utterly delicious and a perfect dessert for the keto diet.

SERVING SIZE:

This recipe yields 8 servings.

INGREDIENTS:

Fudge:

1/2 cup peanut butter

1/4 cup butter (melted)

1/2 tsp. vanilla extract

1/4 cup heavy cream

1/4 cup erythritol

1/8 tsp xanthan gum

Crust:

1 tbsp. erythritol

1/4 cup butter (melted)

1 cup almond flour

1/2 tsp. cinnamon

1 pinch salt

Topping:

1/3 cup dark chocolate (chopped)

DIRECTIONS:

1. Preheat your oven to 400°F.

2. Combine all of the ingredients for the crust, and mix thoroughly.

3. When smooth, line a baking dish with parchment paper and press the mixture into the bottom.

4. Bake for 10 minutes, and let cool.

5. Blend all the fudge ingredients with a food processor or blender. Now spread the fudge over the baked crust.

6. Top with the chopped chocolate and chill overnight.

Savor the sweetness!

NUTRITIONAL INFORMATION (PER SERVING):

Calories: 302

Fat: 19.5g

Carbs: 4g

Protein: 5g

Buttered Pecan Ice Cream

Yet another gloriously keto friendly ice cream version! Enjoy this mouthwatering combination of browned butter, coconut, and pecans!

Serving size:

This recipe yields 4 servings.

Ingredients:

5 tbsp. butter

1/4 tsp. xanthan gum

1 1/2 cups coconut milk (unsweetened)

25 drops liquid stevia

1/4 cup heavy cream

1/4 cup pecans (crushed)

DIRECTIONS:

1. Heat a pan on low, and add the butter. Heat until the butter turns amber.

2. Toss in the stevia, pecans, and cream. Stir continuously until well combined.

3. Now mix in the gum and milk.

4. Pour into your ice cream maker and follow the churning instructions.

Enjoy!

NUTRITIONAL INFORMATION (PER SERVING):

Calories: 315

Fat: 35g

Carbs: 1.5g

Protein: 0.5g

KETO MUG CHURRO

Churros in mug form! The same wonderful combination of vanilla, nutmeg, and cinnamon; but all combined in a mug and ready in seconds!

SERVING SIZE:

This recipe yields 1 serving.

INGREDIENTS:

1/4 tsp cinnamon

1 tbsp. erythritol

1/4 tsp. vanilla

1/4 tsp. nutmeg

1/2 tsp. baking powder

7 drops stevia

1/8 tsp. ginger

4 tbsp. almond flour

1/8 tsp. allspice

2 tbsp. butter

1 egg

DIRECTIONS:

1. Add all ingredients to a mug and mix completely.

2. Microwave on high for 60 to 70 seconds.

3. Tap the mug against and plate and the cake will fall out.

Into your face they go!

Nutritional information (per serving):

Calories: 435

Fat: 43g

Carbs: 5g

Protein: 11g

BUTTERSCOTCH ICE CREAM

Mmm butterscotch ice cream. Creamy, succulent, and keto friendly. With a dash of vodka for an added kick!

SERVING SIZE:
This recipe yields 3 servings.

INGREDIENTS:
3 tbsp. butter (browned)

25 drops liquid stevia

1/4 cup heavy cream

1/2 tsp. xanthan gum

2 tbsp. vodka

2 tsp. butterscotch flavoring

2 tbsp. erythritol

1/4 cup sour cream

1 cup coconut milk

1 tsp. sea salt

DIRECTIONS:

1. If not already done, brown your butter on low heat.

2. Blend all of the ingredients with a food processor, blender, or immersion blender.

3. Pour the mixture into your ice cream maker and follow instructions.

Enjoy!

NUTRITIONAL INFORMATION (PER SERVING):

Calories: 250

Fat: 23g

Carbs: 2.5g

Protein: 1g

MOCHA ICE CREAM

Give your ice cream a little dash of coffee to develop a deep mocha flavor; and combined with coconut milk and cocoa this ice cream is a winner.

SERVING SIZE:

This recipe yields 2 servings.

INGREDIENTS:

2 tbsp. erythritol

15 drops liquid stevia

1 tbsp. instant coffee

1 cup coconut milk

1/4 cup heavy cream

2 tbsp. cocoa powder

1/4 tsp. xanthan gum

DIRECTIONS:

1. Thoroughly blend all ingredients, except for the gum, in a blender or food processor.

2. Blend on lowest setting and slowly add the xanthan gum.

3. Pour the mixture into your ice cream machine and follow manufacturer's instructions.

Eat to your heart's content.

NUTRITIONAL INFORMATION (PER SERVING):

Calories: 143

Fat: 15.5g

Carbs: 2g

Protein: 1.5g

Coconutty Chocolate Macaroons

The combination of chocolate and coconut is a tried and true dessert favorite. Try our coconutty chocolate macaroons and find out for yourself!

SERVING SIZE:

This recipe yields 20 servings.

INGREDIENTS:

1/3 cup coconut (shredded and unsweetened)

3 tbsp. coconut flour

1/4 cup coconut oil

1 tsp. vanilla extract

1/2 tsp. baking powder

1 cup almond flour

2 large eggs

1/3 cup erythritol

1/4 tsp. salt

1/4 cup cocoa powder

DIRECTIONS:

1. Preheat your oven to 350°F.

2. Thoroughly mix all dry ingredients.

3. Now slowly add all the wet ingredients, while stirring continuously.

4. Use your hand to roll out the balls and place on a greased baking sheet.

5. Bake for 15 to 20 minutes

Share the love!

NUTRITIONAL INFORMATION (PER SERVING):

Calories: 75

Fat: 7g

Carbs: 1.5g

Protein: 2.5g

KETO COOKIE BUTTER

Keto cookie butter? Oh yes, it does exist. Oh recipe is perfect for spreading on bread, or other desserts, or eating by the spoonful!

SERVING SIZE:

This recipe is good for 16 servings.

INGREDIENTS:

2 tbsp. butter

1/8 tsp. nutmeg

1 tsp. vanilla

2 tbsp. heavy cream

1/8 tsp. cloves

1/4 tsp. ginger

1/4 tsp cinnamon

2 tbsp. swerve sweetener

1 cup macadamias

3/4 cup cashews

1 pinch salt

DIRECTIONS:

1. Add all the nuts to a food processor and pulse until smooth.

2. Heat a pan on medium and brown your butter. Mix in the swerve.

3. Now add the heavy cream and stir. Remove from heat and add to nut mixture in food processor.

4. Toss in the vanilla and all spices. Continue to process and make sure no lumps remain.

5. Process until you get your desired consistency.

Enjoy!

NUTRITIONAL INFORMATION (PER SERVING):

Calories: 112

Fat: 12g

1.5g

Protein: 2g

PEANUT BUTTER MILKSHAKE

This milkshake has only a few ingredients and will definitely help you satisfy that peanut butter craving. You can also tailor any of the ingredients until you get a shake that's your perfect fit! See our next recipe for strawberry milkshake to see how easy it is to customize this recipe.

SERVING SIZE:

This recipe yields 1 serving.

INGREDIENTS:

2 tbsp. Sugar free caramel syrup (such as SF Torani)

7 ice cubes

1 tbsp. MCT oil

1/4 tsp. xanthan gum

1 cup coconut milk

2 tbsp. peanut butter

DIRECTIONS:

1. Toss all of your ingredients into a blender, and blend until you get your desired consistency.

2. You can tailor the amount of ingredients until you get the taste and consistency you want.

Simple as that, really!

NUTRITIONAL INFORMATION (PER SERVING):

Calories: 365

Fat: 36g

Carbs: 5.5g

Protein: 7.5g

STRAWBERRY MILKSHAKE

Here's a variation on the peanut butter milkshake. Same base ingredients of coconut milk, MCT oil, and xanthan gum for the base, but you can always tailor your flavoring!

SERVING SIZE:

This recipe yields 1 serving:

INGREDIENTS:

2 tbsp. Sugar free strawberry syrup (such as SF Torani)

7 ice cubes

1 tbsp. MCT oil

1/4 tsp. xanthan gum

3/4 cup coconut milk

1/4 cup heavy cream

DIRECTIONS:

1. Toss all of your ingredients into a blender, and blend until you get your desired consistency.

2. You can tailor the amount of ingredients until you get the taste and consistency you want.

Enjoy!

Nutritional information (per serving):

Calories: 375

Fat: 42g

Carbs: 2.5g

Protein: 0g

CHUNKY CHOCOLATE ICE CREAM

The classic chocolate chunk ice cream, but keto friendly! Perfect for those warm evenings with avocados for added creaminess!

SERVING SIZE:

This recipe yields 6 servings

INGREDIENTS:

1/2 cup erythritol (powdered)

1/2 cup heavy cream

1/2 cup cocoa powder

1 cup coconut milk

2 tsp. vanilla extract

25 drops liquid stevia

6 squares baker's chocolate (unsweetened)

2 ripe avocados

DIRECTIONS:

1. Peel and remove the pits from your avocados. Add to a bowl along with the vanilla, milk, and cream.

2. Use an immersion blender until you have a uniform, creamy, mixture. A food processor would also work here.

3. Now toss in your cocoa powder, erythritol, and stevia.

4. Make sure everything is completely mixed then add the chopped chocolate to the bowl.

5. Refrigerate the mixture for at least 10 hours. Then add to ice cream maker and follow instructions.

Go get it!

NUTRITIONAL INFORMATION (PER SERVING):

Calories: 240

Fat: 22.5g

Carbs: 4g

Protein: 4g

CHIA SEED BLONDIES

Chia seeds make an excellent thickening agent for baking, and they're on the keto diet's side. Try out this blondie recipe using ground chia seeds and see for yourself!

SERVING SIZE:

This recipe yields 16 servings.

INGREDIENTS:

3 large eggs

1/4 cup erythritol (powdered)

3 tbsp. Sugar free salted caramel sauce (SF torani)

10 drops liquid stevia

1 tsp. baking powder

1/2 cup chia seeds (ground)

2 1/4 cups pecans (roasted)

3 tbsp. heavy cream

1 pinch salt

1/4 cup butter (melted)

DIRECTIONS:

1. Preheat oven to 350°F

2. Bake your pecans for about 10 minutes

3. Grind the erythritol and chia seeds in a food processor until a powder is formed.

4. Now add 2/3 of your pecans to a food processor (alone) and processor until a butter forms.

5. Toss in the stevia, salt, eggs, salt, and chia/erythritol. Mix well

6. Chop the remaining pecans, and add the rest of the ingredients to the batter. Mix well.

7. Place in a greased 9x9 baking pan and bake for 20 minutes.

Let cool and serve!

NUTRITIONAL INFORMATION (PER SERVING):

Calories: 175

Fat: 17g

Carbs: 1.5g

Protein: 4g

COCONUT MOCHA MUG CAKE

Another quick, single serving, mug cake. Featuring a blend of coconut and mocha, this mug cake is a relaxing end to your day or a perfect midday snack!

SERVING SIZE:

This recipe yields 1 serving.

INGREDIENTS:

1 tbsp. cocoa powder

1/2 tsp. instant coffee

1 large egg

7 drops liquid stevia

1 tbsp. erythritol

1 tbsp. coconut milk

1 tbsp. shredded coconut (unsweetened)

2 tsp. coconut flour

2 tbsp. almond flour

1/2 tsp. baking powder

2 tbsp. butter

DIRECTIONS:

1. Add all ingredients to a mug and mix completely.

2. Microwave on high for 65 to 75 seconds.

3. Tap the mug against and plate and the cake will fall out.

Done!

NUTRITIONAL INFORMATION (PER SERVING):

Calories: 415

Fat: 39g

Carbs: 5g

Protein: 10.5g

GREENIE LATTE

Ginger! Allspice! Vanilla! And many more delicious ingredients make up this latte. Whip it up after dinner for a soothing evening and enjoy!

SERVING SIZE:

This recipe yields 2 servings.

INGREDIENTS:

1/2 tsp. cinnamon

3/4 cup coconut milk

1/4 tsp. allspice

1/4 tsp. ginger

2 tbsp. butter

1 cup strong brewed coffee

1/4 tsp. cardamom

2 tbsp. erythritol

1/2 tsp. vanilla extract

2 handfuls spinach

1/2 cup pumpkin puree

2 handfuls ice

10 drops liquid stevia

DIRECTIONS:

1. Add all of the ingredients to a blender or food processor and mix well.

2. Top with some extra cinnamon or homemade whipped cream if you like!

How easy was that?

NUTRITIONAL INFORMATION (PER SERVING):

Calories: 150

Fat: 14g

Carbs: 4g

Protein: 3g

Whiskey Vanilla Mug Cake

Mug cakes are an easy and fast antidote for a sweet tooth, and they can be keto friendly too! Try out this boozy version with some whiskey for an added boost!

Serving Size:

This recipe yields 1 serving.

Ingredients:

7 drops stevia

3 tbsp. almond flour

2 tbsp. butter

1 tbsp. erythritol

1 tbsp. whiskey

2 tsp. coconut flour

1/2 tsp. vanilla extract

1/2 tsp. baking powder

1 egg

DIRECTIONS:

1. Add all ingredients to a mug and mix completely.

2. Microwave on high for 80 to 90 seconds.

3. Tap the mug against and plate and the cake will fall out.

Enjoy!

NUTRITIONAL INFORMATION (PER SERVING):

Calories: 445

Fat: 41g

Carbs: 4.5g

Protein: 12.5g

Chocolate Peanut Butter Mug Cake

Yet another combination of peanut butter and chocolate! This time in the form of another mug cake. Made with almond flour and butter, this is a perfect dessert without torpedoing your keto diet!

Serving size:

This recipe yields 1 serving.

Ingredients:

2 tbsp. almond flour

1/2 tsp. vanilla

1 tbsp. erythritol

10g dark chocolate

7 drops stevia

1 large egg

1 tbsp. peanut butter

1/2 tsp. baking powder

2 tbsp. butter

DIRECTIONS:

1. Add all ingredients to a mug and mix completely.

2. Microwave on high for 60 to 70 seconds.

3. Tap the mug against and plate and the cake will fall out.

Enjoy!

NUTRITIONAL INFORMATION (PER SERVING):

Calories: 490

Fat: 48g

Carbs: 4.5g

Protein: 13.5g

MAPLE MUG CAKE

Get the delicious taste of maple in your dessert with this mug cake. Wonderfully easy to make and you'll be enjoying it in no time!

SERVING SIZE:
This recipe yields 1 serving.

INGREDIENTS:
2 tbsp. almond flour

1/2 tsp. maple extract

2 tbsp. butter

2 tbsp. crushed pecans

7 drops stevia

1/2 tsp. baking powder

1/4 tsp. cinnamon

1 tbsp. erythritol

1 large egg

DIRECTIONS:

1. Add all ingredients to a mug and mix completely.

2. Microwave on high for 55 to 60 seconds.

3. Tap the mug against and plate and the cake will fall out.

Eat!

NUTRITIONAL INFORMATION (PER SERVING):

Calories: 435

Fat: 45g

Carbs: 3g

Protein: 10.5g

CHOCOLATE MUG CAKE

Classic chocolate brownie, in a mug, ready in seconds! Whip it up and enjoy this dessert staple.

SERVING SIZE:

This recipe yields 2 servings.

INGREDIENTS:

2 tsp. coconut flour

2 tbsp. butter (melted, salted)

2 tbsp. almond flour

1/2 tsp. baking powder

1 1/2 tbsp. erythritol

1/4 tsp. vanilla extract

1 large egg

2 tbsp. cocoa powder

DIRECTIONS:

1. Add all ingredients to a mug and mix completely.

2. Microwave on high for 65 to 70 seconds.

3. Tap the mug against and plate and the cake will fall out.

Simple, no?

Nutritional information (per serving):

Calories: 195

Fat: 20g

Carbs: 3g

Protein: 5.5g

KETO CHOCOLATE GANACHE

Here's a straightforward, keto style, chocolate ganache that can be used for any dessert! Try spreading it over some mug brownies, or coconut bars, or whatever chocolate goes with (which is basically everything).

SERVING SIZE:

This will be enough to cover the goodies we've made so far!

INGREDIENTS:

2 tbsp. heavy cream

1 1/2 oz. chocolate

DIRECTIONS:

1. Boil some water in a pot.

2. Place your chocolate and put it on top of the boiling water to melt it.

3. Once fully melted, add the cream and mix

Ahh, lovely!

NUTRITIONAL INFORMATION:

Calories: 323

Fat: 24g

Carbs: 5g

Protein: 3g

KETO CHOCOLATE

Ever wanted to make your own homemade chocolate? Well here you go! Just a few ingredients and it's all yours!

SERVING SIZE:

This recipe yields 24 servings.

INGREDIENTS:

2/3 cup LC-natural sweet white

1 cup expeller pressed coconut oil

1 cup cocoa powder

DIRECTIONS:

1. Add oil to bowl and melt over a hot pan of water (don't let the bowl touch the water).

2. Combine the cocoa and sweetener in a bowl and mix completely.

3. When oil is melted, add to cocoa mixture and mix thoroughly.

4. Cool, or chill in the fridge, until it reaches your desired consistency.

Enjoy!

NUTRITIONAL INFORMATION (PER SERVING):

Calories: 100

Fat: 9.5g

Carbs: 1g

Protein: 1g

KETO HOT CHOCOLATE

Those cold and rainy evenings can be improved immeasurably by some hot chocolate. Here we have a keto save recipe that will warm you to the core!

SERVING SIZE:

This recipe yields 2 servings.

INGREDIENTS:

1/2 tsp. vanilla extract

2 tbsp. heavy cream

1 tsp. instant coffee

1 tbsp. Splenda

1/2 tsp. cinnamon

2 tbsp. cocoa powder (unsweetened)

1 1/2 cups coconut milk (unsweetened)

DIRECTIONS:

1. Heat a pan on medium and add the heavy cream and milk.

2. When the mixture starts to steam, add the coffee and cinnamon. Mix well

3. Now add the cocoa powder, and mix again.

4. Toss in the Splenda and vanilla, stir again and make sure no lumps are forming.

5. Now turn up the heat to high, and stir constantly until a rolling boil develops.

6. Once it begins to boil, turn down the heat and keep stirring.

When cooled to your desired level, serve it up!

NUTRITIONAL INFORMATION (PER SERVING):

Calories: 105

Fat: 9.5g

Carbs: 3.5g

Protein: 1g

PEANUT BUTTER AND CHOCOLATE PUDDING

Oh, chocolate and peanut butter, why are you so amazing together? If you need any further proof that these two may just be the best combination ever for dessert, try this pudding!

SERVING SIZE:

This recipe yields 1 serving.

INGREDIENTS:

1 tsp. cocoa powder

1/4 tsp. allspice

2 tbsp. peanut butter

5 drops liquid stevia

1 tbsp. coconut oil

1 tbsp. heavy cream

DIRECTIONS:

1. Combine all of the ingredients in a cup or mug and stir completely, making sure there are no lumps.

2. Freeze for a couple hours.

Pull out of the freezer and dive in!

NUTRITIONAL INFORMATION:

Calories: 386

Fat: 8g

Carbs: 4.5g

Protein: 7.5g

MUSCLE CHOCOLATE CAKE

Want a little protein boost while still enjoying dessert? Then whip up this chocolate mug cake made with a scoop of protein powder!

SERVING SIZE:

This recipe yields 1 serving:

INGREDIENTS:

1 scoop protein powder

2 large eggs

1 tbsp. heavy cream

1 packet Splenda

DIRECTIONS:

1. Add all of the ingredients to a mug and mix completely.

2. Microwave for about 1 minute, check, and microwave longer if you wish.

Go for it!

NUTRITIONAL INFORMATION:

Calories: 310

Fat: 15.5g

Carbs: 4.5g

Protein: 37g

CHOCOLATE PEANUT BUTTER ICE CREAM

Yet another combination of peanut butter and chocolate. Try this unique ice cream recipe incorporating cottage cheese for creaminess and protein powder!

SERVING SIZE:
This recipe yields 2 servings.

INGREDIENTS:
6 drops Splenda

2 tbsp. peanut butter

1 cup cottage cheese

1 scoop protein powder

2 tbsp. heavy cream

DIRECTIONS:

1. Combine the cheese and Splenda in a food processor.

2. Toss in the peanut butter and cream. Blend well.

3. Keep blending until all the cheese curds are smooth.

4. Now add the protein powder and blend again.

5. Freeze for at least an hour and enjoy!

NUTRITIONAL INFORMATION (PER SERVING):

Calories: 335

Fat: 18.5g

Carbs: 6g

Protein: 30.5g

KETO MUG BROWNIE

Chocolate mug brownie, plain and simple. Whip it up in seconds, enjoy, and repeat as required!

SERVING SIZE:

This recipe yields 1 serving.

INGREDIENTS:

1 tsp. cocoa powder

1 pinch baking soda

1 tbsp. egg white (beaten)

1 tbsp. almond butter

1/8 tsp. vanilla extract

3 drops stevia

1 pinch salt

DIRECTIONS:

1. Add all ingredients to a mug and mix completely.

2. Microwave on high for 50 seconds.

3. Tap the mug against and plate and the cake will fall out.

Knock it back, you deserve it!

NUTRITIONAL INFORMATION (PER SERVING):

Calories: 104

Fat: 8.5g

Carbs: 3g

Protein: 5g

KETO WHITE CHOCOLATE BARK

This deliciously smooth white chocolate bark makes an excellent dessert to have on hand in the fridge, or for taking to an event.

SERVING SIZE:

This recipe yields 12 servings.

INGREDIENTS:

1/2 tsp. hemp seed powder

1/3 cup LC-Natural sweet white

2 oz. cacao butter

1 tsp. vanilla powder

1 tsp. pumpkin seeds (toasted)

1 pinch salt

DIRECTIONS:

1. Melt the butter in a bowl over hot water, and make sure the bowl doesn't touch the water.

2. Mix all ingredients with the butter once it is melted.

3. Pour the mixture into a greased baking dish.

4. All the mixture time to set and firm up.

5. Placing in the freezer will also help speed up the setting process.

Yum, enjoy!

NUTRITIONAL INFORMATION (PER SERVING):

Calories: 40

Fat: 2g

Carbs: 0g

Protein: 0g

CHAI MUG CAKE

Chai tea is renowned for its soothing properties. So why not bring that over to a dessert! Try this blend of relaxing spices combined in a delectable brownie.

SERVING SIZE:

This recipe yields 1 serving.

INGREDIENTS:

4 tbsp. almond flour

7 drops stevia

1/4 tsp. cloves

1/4 tsp. cinnamon

1/4 tsp. vanilla

1/2 tsp. baking powder

1 tbsp. erythritol

2 tbsp. butter

1/4 tsp. cardamom

1/4 tsp. ginger

1 large egg

DIRECTIONS:

1. Add all ingredients to a mug and mix completely.

2. Microwave on high for 65 to 70 seconds.

3. Tap the mug against and plate and the cake will fall out.

All done and ready to eat!

NUTRITIONAL INFORMATION (PER SERVING):

Calories: 440

Fat: 44g

Carbs: 3.5g

Protein: 12.5g

MACADAMIA COCONUT CUSTARD

Nutty macadamia custard made in coconut milk to give it fantastic taste! We recommend chilling in the fridge overnight, so plan ahead with this one!

SERVING SIZE:

This recipe yields 4 servings.

INGREDIENTS:

1/3 cup macadamia nut butter

1 tsp. liquid stevia

1/3 cup heavy cream

1/3 cup erythritol

1 tsp. vanilla extract

4 large eggs

1 cup coconut milk (unsweetened)

DIRECTIONS:

1. Preheat your oven to 325°F.

2. Combine all of your ingredients in a bowl. Whisk well to make sure everything is combined.

3. Pour about 1 inch of water into the bottom of a baking dish and place four ramekins in the dish (the water should come about halfway up the sides)

4. Fill the ramekins with your mixture.

5. Bake for about 40 minutes. A knife will come out of the center clean when the custard is cooked.

6. Cool for half an hour.

That's it, good to go!

NUTRITIONAL INFORMATION (PER SERVING):

Calories: 272

Fat: 26g

Carbs: 3g

Protein: 6g

"A crust eaten in peace is better than a banquet partaken in anxiety."

-Aesop

FREE BONUS GUIDE:
TOP 10 KETO DIET MISTAKES

We hope you enjoy making your way through the delicious meals contained in this cookbook.

To ensure you stay safe and maximize your progress be sure to pick up your free bonus guide below now to avoid the top 10 keto diet mistakes!

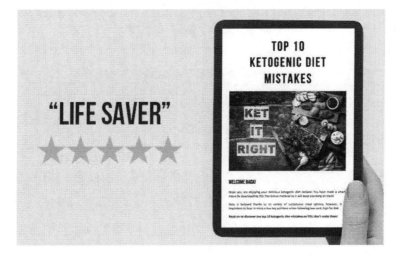

Visit www.litomedia.com/ketogenic-mistakes to get your free bonus guide!

LIKE THIS BOOK?

If you enjoyed the meals in this cookbook, please visit your Amazon order history to leave a review and let us know.

If you also downloaded the free bonus guide, you will know the value of community, so don't forget to share this book with a friend too!

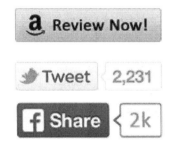

58540148R00078

Made in the USA
San Bernardino, CA
29 November 2017